THE WISDOM OF MY SKELETAL SYSTEM

How Exercise And Nutrition Impact Bone Health

BY

Jose A. Smith

Copyright © 2023 by Jose A. Smith All rights reserved. No part of this publication may be reproduced, stored or transmitted in any form or by any means, electronic, mechanical, photocopying, recording, scanning, or otherwise without written permission from the publisher. It is illegal to copy this book, post it to a website, or distribute it by any other means without permission.

TABLE OF CONTENTS

CHAPTER 1..*5*

   INTRODUCTION TO BONE HEALTH 5

CHAPTER 2..*11*

   THE IMPORTANCE OF EXERCISE FOR BONE HEALTH........................11

CHAPTER 3..*16*

   THE IMPACT OF NUTRITION ON BONE HEALTH...............................16

CHAPTER 4..*21*

CHAPTER 5..*25*

   DIAGNOSING AND TREATING BONE HEALTH PROBLEMS 25

CHAPTER 6..*30*

   CONCLUSION AND RECOMMENDATIONS 30

CHAPTER 1

INTRODUCTION TO BONE HEALTH

A crucial component of overall health and fitness is bone health. The state of the bones in the human body, including its strength, density, and capacity to sustain the body and safeguard its internal organs, is referred to as the term's definition. The mobility, stability, and quality of life of an individual, as well as their capacity to carry out everyday tasks and retain independence, are all impacted by their bone health.

The skeletal system is an essential part of the human body because it helps bones perform their protective function while also giving the body structure and support.

Additionally, the bones have a role in a number of critical physiological processes, including the development of red blood cells, the storage of minerals, and the control of hormones.

Compact bone, spongy bone, and bone marrow are just a few of the numerous forms of tissue that make up the bones in the human body. While spongy bone is less dense and is found in the center of bones, compact bone is more dense and strong and makes up the outer layer of bones. Blood cells are created in the soft tissue called bone marrow, which is located inside the bones.

The joints, which are specialized regions where two bones meet, hold the bones together. To prevent wear and tear and lessen friction during movement, cartilage and synovial fluid lubricate and cushion the joints.

Numerous elements, including genetics, diet, exercise, and hormonal imbalances, have an impact on bone health. For instance, a person's peak bone mass, or the highest level of bone density they will ever have in their lifetime, is influenced by genetics. Nutrition is also important because strong bones require a sufficient intake of calcium and vitamin D. In order to increase bone density and prevent osteoporosis, weight-bearing exercises and strength training are important components of a healthy lifestyle. Because estrogen, testosterone, and other hormones are involved in regulating bone metabolism, hormonal imbalances can also affect bone health.

Age is one of the most important variables that determine bone health. People naturally lose bone mass and density as they age, which may result in diseases like osteoporosis and fractures. Bones that have osteoporosis are more prone to become fragile and weak, which increases their risk of breaking. Fractures may cause excruciating pain, severe disability, and a loss of freedom. It is impossible to overestimate the significance of maintaining excellent bone health since it has an impact on many facets of life. Osteoporosis and fractures may be avoided with good bone health, which also lowers the risk of accidents and improves quality of life. Additionally, maintaining excellent bone health might aid in delaying the development of other disorders including osteoarthritis, a degenerative joint disease that damages joint cartilage.

In summary, bone health is an important component of overall health and wellbeing and is impacted by a variety of variables, such as genetics, diet, physical activity, and hormone imbalances. The skeletal system is essential to the functioning of the human body because it offers protection, structure, and support for a number of critical physiological functions. Osteoporosis, fractures, and other problems may be avoided with proper bone health, which can also enhance quality of life. It's crucial to partake in weight-bearing workouts, strength training, and a nutritious diet that contains enough calcium and vitamin D to support strong bones.

CHAPTER 2

THE IMPORTANCE OF EXERCISE FOR BONE HEALTH

Exercise is essential for keeping strong, healthy bones and is also necessary for general health and fitness. The basis of our body is made up of bones, which support and shield our muscles and internal organs. Bones are also crucial to our movement and capacity for everyday tasks. We will discuss the value of exercise for bone health in this chapter, as well as how it may enhance bone health, the kinds of exercises that are most effective for doing so, and the relevance of exercise at various stages of life.

Increased bone density is one of the most well-known advantages of exercise for bones. This is crucial for older people because as they age, their bone density gradually declines, increasing their risk of osteoporosis and fractures. By exerting strain on the bones, weight-bearing workouts like walking, running, or stair climbing serve to enhance bone density. By encouraging the creation of new bone tissue, this force makes bones stronger and more fracture-resistant.

Strength training, such as weightlifting, is another resistance workout that is good for the bones. Resistance training may enhance overall bone strength and promote bone density by pushing the bones to their limits with heavy weights. These workouts serve to maintain the form and alignment of bones while also having a good effect on bone structure. This is crucial for preserving balance and lowering the risk of fractures and falls, particularly in older persons.

Exercise may enhance bone quality in addition to boosting bone density. This relates to the tiny structure of bones, often known as their microarchitecture. Exercise has been demonstrated to increase the amount of microcracks in bones, which helps to develop a more durable structure, thereby improving bone quality. This is crucial for older people because osteoporotic fractures are greatly influenced by poor bone quality.

In addition to having a good effect on bone metabolism, exercise also helps to maintain a healthy balance between bone creation and bone resorption (the process by which new bone tissue is created). Exercise has been found to assist control bone metabolism, which reduces bone loss and improves overall bone health. This balance is essential for keeping healthy bones.

Exercise is crucial for bone health not just in maturity but also in the first years of life. Exercise may significantly affect the creation of strong, healthy bones in children and teens, who are in a crucial stage of bone growth and development. Jumping, jogging, and participating in sports are weight-bearing activities that are particularly beneficial for kids because they support bone growth and development. Resistance training may also increase muscle mass, which can improve bone health overall by lowering the risk of fractures and falls.

In order to preserve bone health in older persons, exercise is crucial. Exercise may assist to lower the risk of fractures in older people since their bones are more brittle and prone to breakage. Exercises that include weight-bearing and resistance may assist to maintain or increase bone density, as well as enhance balance and lower the risk of falling. This is crucial for older people since falls are a leading cause of fractures and may seriously impair mobility and general health.

In conclusion, exercise is essential for keeping strong, healthy bones in addition to being necessary for general health and fitness. For children, teens, and older individuals in particular, weight-bearing and resistance activities are crucial because they help enhance bone quality, density, and metabolism. Making exercise a regular habit can assist to support strong bones and lower your risk of fractures and other associated disorders. Decide on a range of weight-bearing and resistance exercises.

CHAPTER 3

THE IMPACT OF NUTRITION ON BONE HEALTH

Given that bones support the body and shield vital organs, bone health is crucial to overall health and wellbeing. Maintaining strong, healthy bones requires proper nutrition, and certain nutrients are especially crucial for bone health. This chapter will outline the nutrients that are crucial for bone health, go over how diet can impact bone strength and density, and show how to make sure you're getting enough nutrients to maintain good bone health.

Important Foods for Bone Health

The most well-known nutrient for bone health is calcium, which is essential for both the development and upkeep of strong bones. Adults should consume 1000–1300 mg of calcium daily, which can be found in dairy products, leafy green vegetables, and fortified foods like orange juice and tofu.

Because it facilitates calcium absorption and maintains adequate calcium levels in the body, vitamin D is also crucial for bone health. Adults should consume 600–800 IU of vitamin D daily, and foods like fatty fish, egg yolks, and fortified milk and cereal are excellent sources of this vitamin. The body's synthesis of vitamin D is also aided by exposure to the sun.

Because it supplies the building blocks for bone tissue and aids in maintaining bone mass, protein is also crucial for the health of the bones. Lean meats, dairy products, and plant-based sources like beans and nuts are good sources of protein. Adults should consume 0.8 grams of protein per kilogram of body weight per day.

Magnesium, phosphorus, and vitamins K and C are additional crucial elements for bone health. Nuts, seeds, and leafy green vegetables are excellent sources of magnesium, which aids in regulating the body's calcium balance. As it aids in bone formation and maintenance, phosphorus is also crucial for bone health. Meats, poultry, and dairy products are good sources of phosphorus. Leafy green vegetables, vegetable oils, and fermented dairy products are excellent sources of vitamin K, which is necessary for the development and upkeep of bone structure. Citrus fruits, berries, and leafy green vegetables are rich sources of vitamin C, which is necessary for the synthesis of collagen, which strengthens and supports bones.

Diet's effect on bone strength and density

Diet may have a big effect on bone strength and density. Reduced bone density and an increased risk of osteoporosis may result from a diet that is deficient in calcium and other vital elements for healthy bones. Additionally, certain diets and lifestyle choices, like smoking and drinking too much alcohol, may be detrimental to bone health.

Contrarily, a diet high in calcium and other bone-friendly minerals may assist to preserve strong, healthy bones and lower the risk of osteoporosis. Given that bone density always declines with age, this may be particularly crucial for elderly persons. The pace of bone loss may be slowed down and bone density and strength can be maintained with enough calcium intake and other important nutrients.

Making Sure You Get Enough Nutrients for the Best Bone Health

In order to keep strong, healthy bones throughout life, it's crucial to ensure proper nutritional consumption. Eating a well-balanced diet that includes a range of foods from all food categories is one strategy to guarantee appropriate nutrient intake. Additionally, soda and other sugar-sweetened beverages, as well as excessive quantities of alcohol and caffeine, may have a deleterious effect on bone health and should be avoided.

For people who struggle to get enough of certain necessary nutrients via food alone.

CHAPTER 4

COMMON RISK FACTORS FOR BONE LOSS AND FRACTURE

People of all ages are concerned about bone loss and fractures. Age, genetics, lifestyle choices, and underlying medical issues are just a few of the variables that might make these illnesses more likely. It is essential to comprehend the typical causes of bone loss and fracture in order to maintain excellent bone health and avoid associated medical problems.

Age is one of the major risk factors for bone loss and fracture. As individuals age, their bones gradually weaken and are more prone to breaking. This is brought on by the aging-related decrease in bone density, which makes bones more fragile and prone to fracture. Due to hormonal changes that may result in a sudden decrease in bone density, postmenopausal women are especially vulnerable to bone loss.

Genetics is another element that may raise the risk of bone loss and fracture. Some folks are just genetically predisposed to having weak bones. A lack of exercise and bad diet are two lifestyle variables that may make this hereditary susceptibility worse.

Bone health may be significantly impacted by lifestyle choices as well. For instance, sedentary behavior might result in brittle bones and a higher risk of fracture. On the other hand, exercise, particularly weight-bearing sports like running, leaping, and weightlifting, aids in the development and maintenance of strong bones. Fractures and bone loss may also be caused by a diet that is deficient in calcium and vitamin D.

The risk of bone loss and fractures might also be increased by medical problems. For instance, thyroid-related diseases like hyperthyroidism may accelerate bone turnover, which might result in weaker bones. The risk of bone loss may also be increased by ailments such rheumatoid arthritis, osteoporosis, and osteopenia.

CHAPTER 5

DIAGNOSING AND TREATING BONE HEALTH PROBLEMS

From mild disorders like osteoporosis to more serious concerns like fractures and malignancies, there are many different types of bone health problems. In order to get the best results, it is essential to identify and treat bone health problems early on. Maintaining strong bones is essential to ensure general health and mobility.

X-rays, magnetic resonance imaging (MRI), computed tomography (CT) scans, and bone mineral density tests are often used to identify issues with bone health. Especially in situations of suspected fractures or malignancies, X-rays are often employed as the first diagnostic technique. They may demonstrate the presence of a fracture or the thinness and fragility of the bones, which are signs of osteoporosis. Detailed pictures of the bones and surrounding tissues are provided by MRI and CT scans, enabling a more complete assessment of the disease. Dual-energy X-ray absorptiometry (DXA) scans, commonly known as bone mineral density examinations, are used to evaluate bone density and detect whether a person has osteoporosis or is at risk of getting the disease. Conditions that impair bone health may be treated in a number of ways, including with medication, dietary modifications, and in extreme situations, surgery. Bisphosphonates, which slow down bone deterioration, and hormone treatment, which may assist post-menopausal women maintain bone density, are two medications for bone health issues. In order to maintain healthy bones, doctors often prescribe calcium and vitamin D supplements.

A nutritious diet and regular exercise are only two examples of lifestyle modifications that are crucial for preserving bone health. Weight-bearing workouts like running, weightlifting, and walking may support the development and maintenance of strong bones. A well-balanced diet low in sodium and caffeine, high in calcium and Vitamin D, may also support the maintenance of strong bones.

Surgery may be required to address severe instances of bone health issues. For instance, surgery may be necessary to realign the bones and encourage healing when a fracture is not mending correctly. Reconstructive surgery may be required to restore mobility and function in circumstances when tumors or other disorders necessitate the removal of a section of the bone.

It is impossible to stress the significance of early identification and treatment for the best results. For instance, osteoporosis may be identified early and treated to reduce the risk of fractures and other severe effects. To delay the condition's course and lower the risk of fractures, lifestyle modifications and drugs may be used. Similar to this, early fracture discovery may aid in avoiding more significant issues including persistent pain, loss of movement, and even disability.

Early intervention may also lessen the risk of long-term bone injury. For instance, timely treatment for osteoporosis may help to stop additional bone loss and lower the risk of fractures. Early intervention in fracture situations may aid in promoting healing and lowering the risk of consequences including persistent pain and loss of mobility.

In conclusion, concerns with bone health may vary from mild ailments to serious disorders that might affect one's general health and mobility. To get the best results, these disorders must be diagnosed and treated. Bone health issues may be found using a variety of diagnostic methods, such as X-rays, MRIs, CT scans, and measurements of bone mineral density. Treatment options include prescription drugs, dietary adjustments, and in extreme circumstances, surgery. For best results and to preserve strong bones, early identification and treatment are essential.

CHAPTER 6
CONCLUSION AND RECOMMENDATIONS

The book "The Essential Guide to Bone Health" offers in-depth guidance on preserving ideal bone health via activity and diet. The book discusses a variety of issues relating to bone health, such as bone form and function, bone density, variables influencing bone health, and methods to stop bone deterioration. The writers provide insightful analysis and helpful guidance for readers looking to enhance their bone health throughout the whole book.

The significance of comprehending the composition and purpose of bones is one of the major topics covered in the book. Bones are intricate structures that have several functions, including supporting the body, defending essential organs, and assisting in movement. They are constructed of living cells and continually redesigned and replaced minerals, such as calcium and phosphorus. Bone resorption, or the process by which old bone tissue is destroyed and replaced by new tissue, must be balanced with bone production to maintain excellent bone health.

Bone density is a crucial component of bone health. Bone mineral content, especially calcium content, is measured by bone density. Our bones naturally lose density as we age, increasing our risk of fractures and other bone-related issues. However, a number of variables, such as genetics, hormone changes, and lifestyle elements like physical activity and diet, may have an impact on bone density.

One of the most important methods to keep strong bones is via physical exercise. Strong bones may be developed and maintained by exercise, particularly weight-bearing exercises. The authors advise include weight-bearing workouts like walking, running, trekking, and resistance training in your program. By putting stress on the bones, these activities aid in promoting bone development by encouraging the body to manufacture new bone tissue. Regular exercise may also assist to enhance general health and lower the chance of developing other illnesses like diabetes and heart disease.

Additionally important to preserving healthy bone health is nutrition. The need of eating a balanced diet that contains enough calcium, phosphorus, vitamin D, and other nutrients is emphasized by the authors. Since calcium is the main mineral that goes into making bones, it is extremely significant. Leafy greens, dairy products, and fortified meals are all excellent sources of calcium. Because it aids in the body's absorption of calcium, vitamin D is especially crucial. Fatty fish, mushrooms, and fortified meals are good sources of vitamin D, as is getting sunshine.

The authors also stress the need of seeing a doctor if you have any concerns regarding your bone health. Bone health may be monitored and possible issues can be identified early on with the use of routine exams and bone density testing. Consult with a healthcare professional if you have any concerns about your bone health so they can help you discover any underlying problems and provide you the right advice. Additionally, it is crucial to take precautions to preserve excellent bone health and seek medical guidance as required if you have a family history of osteoporosis or other bone-related issues.

In conclusion, "The Essential Guide to Bone Health" gives a thorough review of the important variables that influence bone health and offers helpful suggestions for preserving good bone health. The authors stress the need of include exercise and a healthy diet in daily routine as well as seeing a doctor if you have any concerns about your bone health. You can contribute to ensuring that your bones are strong, healthy, and capable of supporting you throughout your life by heeding these advice.

Recommendations include the need for regular weight-bearing activity, a balanced diet rich in calcium, phosphorus, and vitamin D, and seeing a doctor if you have any concerns about your bone health. Additionally, it's important to be aware of lifestyle choices that might harm bone healt

www.ingramcontent.com/pod-product-compliance
Lightning Source LLC
Chambersburg PA
CBHW070321220526
45465CB00013B/2108